Diabetics : Mellitus

Introduction and General discussion

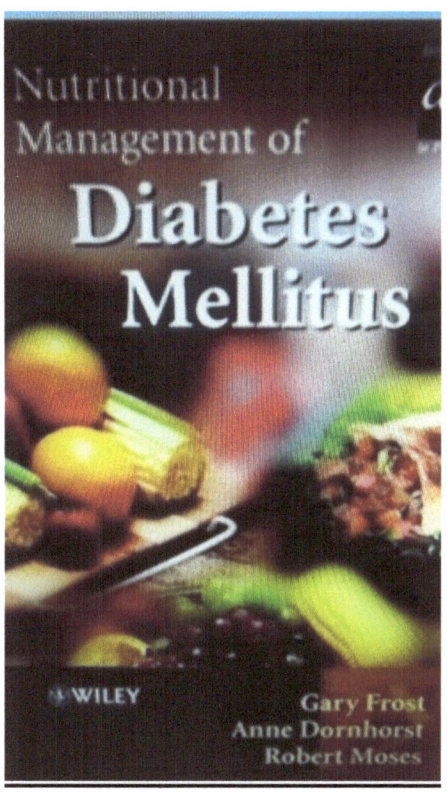

Diabetes mellitus is the world's largest endocrine disorder of multiple etiologies involving metabolic disorders of carbohydrate fat and protein. All forms of diabetes are due to decrease in the circulating concentration of insulin (insulin deficiency) and a decrease in the response of peripheral tissues to insulin (insulin resistance). The aging populations, consumption of calorie-rich diets, obesity and sedentary lifestyles have led to a tremendous increase in the number of individuals with type 2 diabetes worldwide. According to World Health Organization projections, the prevalence of diabetes is likely to increase by 35% by the year 2025. (Boyle *et al.*, 2001)

Diabetes is a serious metabolic disorder with micro- and macro vascular complications that result in significant morbidity and mortality. In the United state diabetes is considered as the third leading cause of death after heart disease and cancer. (Medicinenet.com) Worldwide 177 million people suffer from diabetes. This figure is likely to more than double by 2030. (Databases 4.ht min) Statistical Projections for India suggest that the number of diabetics will rise from 15 million in 1995 to 57 million in the year 2025. (King *et al.*, 1998)

At present the treatment of diabetes mainly involves a sustained reduction in hyperglycaemia (higher amount of sugar in blood) by the use of some drug like biguanides, thiazolidinediones, sulfonylureas D-phenylalanine and α-glucosidase inhibitors in addition to insulin. However, due to unwanted side effects the efficacies of these compounds are debatable and there is a demand for new compounds for the treatment of diabetes. (U.K.PDS, 1995, Moller, 2001) Hence plants have been suggested as a rich, as yet unexplored source of potentially useful antidiabetic drugs. Many traditional plants treatment for diabetes are used throughout the World. Plant drugs and herbal formulations are frequently considered to be less toxic and free from side effects than synthetic one. (Bailey and Day, 1989)

Based on the WHO recommendations hypoglycemic agents of plant origin used in traditional medicine are important. (WHO, 1980) The attributed anti hyperglycemic effects of these plants is due to their ability to restore the function of pancreatic tissues by causing an increase in insulin output or inhibits the intestinal absorption of glucose or to the facilitation of metabolites in insulin dependent processes. Hence, treatment with herbal drugs has an effect on protecting β-cells and smoothing out fluctuation in glucose levels. (Jia *et al.*, 2003) In general there is very little biological knowledge on the specific mode of action in the treatment of diabetes, but most of the plants have been found to contain substances like glycosides, alkaloids, terpenoids, flavonoids etc that are frequently implicated as having antidiabetic effects

Diabetes mellitus is a global metabolic epidemic affecting essential biochemical activities in almost every age group. Indian literatures like Ayurveda have already mentioned herbal remediation for a number of human ailments. Among Indian traditional medicinal plants several potential anti-diabetic plants and herbs are being used as part of our diet since prehistoric time. India has a long list of native medicinal plants with confirmed blood sugar lowering property. Some of these have proved remarkable for cure of diabetes and its complications.

There are several mechanisms through which these herbs act to control the glucose level. They are more or less similar to the actions of synthetic drugs. The mechanism of action of herbal anti-diabetics could be grouped as:

➢ Stimulation of insulin secretion (*Teucrium polium, Allium sativum, Allium cepa, Panic ginseng*)

➢ Inhibition in renal glucose reinsertion (*Fraxinus excelsior*)

➢ Stimulation of glycogenesis and hepatic glycolysis (*Momordica charantia*)

➢ Protective effect on the destruction of the beta-cells (*Thea sinensis*)

➢ Improvement of digestion and reduction of blood sugar and urea (*Aegle marmelos*)

➢ Prevents pathological conversion of starch to glucose (*Eugenia jambolina* and *Pterocarpus marsupium*)

➢ Inhibits β-galactocidase and α-glucocidase (*Clitoria ternata*)

➢ Increasing the use of glucose by tissues and effect on adrenergic receptors (*Panax ginseng, Allium sativum, Allium cepa*)

➢ Potentiates the action of exogenously injected insulin cortisol lowering activities (*Inula racemosa, Boerhaavia diffusa* and *Ocimum sanctum*).

Definition and Classification of Diabetes Mellitus

Definition: Diabetes mellitus is a group of metabolic diseases characterized by hyperglycemia resulting from defects in insulin secretion, insulin action, or both. The chronic hyperglycemia of diabetes is associated with long-term damage, dysfunction, and failure of various organs, especially the eyes, kidneys, nerves, heart, and blood vessels. (*Diabetes Care* 2000 (American Diabetes Association)

Several pathogenic processes are involved in the development of diabetes. These range from autoimmune destruction of the ß-cells of the pancreas with consequent insulin deficiency to abnormalities that result in resistance to insulin action. The basis of the abnormalities in carbohydrate, fat, and protein metabolism in diabetes is deficient action of insulin on target tissues. Deficient insulin action results from inadequate insulin secretion and/or diminished tissue responses to insulin at one or more points in the complex pathways of hormone action.

Classification

The vast majority of cases of diabetes fall into two broad etiopathogenetic categories. In one category,

type 1 diabetes, the cause is an absolute deficiency of insulin secretion. Individuals at increased risk of developing this type of diabetes can often be identified by serological evidence of an autoimmune pathologic process occurring in the pancreatic islets and by genetic markers. In the other, much more prevalent category,

type 2 diabetes, the cause is a combination of resistance to insulin action and an inadequate compensatory insulin secretory response. (Diabetes Care, 1997, 2003)

a) **Type 1 diabetes (ß-cell destruction, usually leading to absolute insulin deficiency):**

   i) **Immune-mediated diabetes-** This form of diabetes, which accounts for only 5–10% of those with diabetes, previously encompassed by the terms insulin-dependent diabetes, type I diabetes, or juvenile-onset diabetes, results from a cellular-mediated autoimmune destruction of the ß-cells of the pancreas.

ii)

In this form of diabetes, the rate of ß-cell destruction is quite variable, being rapid in some individuals (mainly infants and children) and slow in others (mainly adults). Autoimmune destruction of ß-cells has multiple genetic predispositions and is also related to environmental factors that are still poorly defined. Although patients are rarely obese when they present with this type of diabetes, the presence of obesity is not incompatible with the diagnosis. These patients are also prone to other autoimmune disorders such as Graves' disease, Hashimoto's thyroiditis, Addison's disease, vitiligo, celiac sprue, autoimmune hepatitis, myasthenia gravis, and pernicious anemia.

ii) **Idiopathic diabetes-** Some forms of type 1 diabetes has no known etiologies. Some of these patients have permanent insulinopenia and are prone to ketoacidosis. This form of diabetes is strongly inherited, lacks immunological evidence for ß-cell autoimmunity, and is not HLA associated. An absolute requirement for insulin replacement therapy in affected patients may come and go.

b) **Type 2 diabetes:** This form of diabetes, which accounts for 90–95% of those with diabetes, previously referred to as non-insulin-dependent diabetes, type II diabetes, or adult-onset diabetes, encompasses individuals who have insulin resistance and usually have relative (rather than absolute) insulin deficiency At least initially, and often throughout their lifetime, these individuals do not need insulin treatment to survive.

c)

Most patients with this form of diabetes are obese, and obesity itself causes some degree of insulin resistance. Patients who are not obese by traditional weight criteria may have an increased percentage of body fat distributed predominantly in the abdominal region. Ketoacidosis seldom occurs spontaneously in this type of diabetes; when seen, it usually arises in association with the stress of another illness such as infection. Such patients are at increased risk of developing macrovascular and micro vascular complications.

c) **Other specific types of diabetes:**

i) **Genetic defects of the ß-cell- Several forms of diabetes** are associated with monogenetic defects in ß-cell function. These forms of diabetes are frequently characterized by onset of hyperglycemia at an early age (generally before age 25 years. Abnormalities at six genetic loci on different chromosomes have been identified to date. The most common form is associated with mutations on chromosome 12 in a hepatic transcription factor referred to as hepatocyte nuclear factor (HNF)-1. A second form is associated with mutations in the glucokinase gene on chromosome 7p and results in a defective glucokinase molecule. Glucokinase converts glucose to glucose-6-phosphate, the metabolism of which, in turn, stimulates insulin secretion by the ß-cell. The less common forms result from mutations in other transcription factors, including HNF-4, HNF-1ß, insulin promoter factor (IPF)-1, and NeuroD1. Genetic abnormalities that result in the inability to convert proinsulin to insulin have been identified in a few families, and such traits are inherited in an autosomal dominant pattern.

ii) **Genetic defects in insulin action-** The metabolic abnormalities associated with mutations of the insulin receptor may range from hyperinsulinemia and modest hyperglycemia to severe diabetes Leprechaunism and the Rabson-Mendenhall syndrome are two pediatric syndromes that have mutations in the insulin receptor gene with subsequent alterations in insulin receptor function and extreme insulin resistance. The former has characteristic facial features and is usually fatal in infancy, while the latter is associated with abnormalities of teeth and nails and pineal gland hyperplasia.

ii) **Diseases of the exocrine pancreas-** Any process that diffusely injures the pancreas can cause diabetes. Acquired processes include pancreatitis, trauma, infection, pancreatectomy, and pancreatic carcinoma.

iii)

iv) **Endocrinopathies-** Several hormones (e.g., growth hormone, cortisol, glucagon, and epinephrine) antagonize insulin action. Excess amounts of these hormones (e.g., acromegaly, Cushing's syndrome, glucagonoma, pheochromocytoma, respectively) can cause diabetes. This generally occurs in individuals with preexisting defects in insulin secretion.

V) **Drug-** or chemical-induced diabetes- Many drugs can impair insulin secretion. These drugs may not cause diabetes by themselves, but they may precipitate diabetes in individuals with insulin resistance, Examples include nicotinic acid and glucocorticoids. Patients receiving -interferon have been reported to develop diabetes associated with islet cell antibodies and, in certain instances, severe insulin deficiency

vi) **Infections-** Certain viruses have been associated with ß-cell destruction. Diabetes occurs in patients with congenital rubella, although most of these patients have HLA and immune markers characteristic of type 1 diabetes. In addition, coxsackievirus B, cytomegalovirus, adenovirus, and mumps have been implicated in inducing certain cases of the disease.

d) **Gestational diabetes mellitus (GDM):** GDM is defined as any degree of glucose intolerance with onset or first recognition during pregnancy. The definition applies regardless of whether insulin or only diet modification is used for treatment or whether the condition persists after pregnancy. It does not exclude the possibility that unrecognized glucose intolerance may have antedated or begun concomitantly with the pregnancy. GDM complicates 4% of all pregnancies in the U.S., resulting in 135,000 cases annually. The prevalence may range from 1 to 14% of pregnancies, depending on the population studied. GDM represents nearly 90% of all pregnancies complicated by diabetes.

Deterioration of glucose tolerance occurs normally during pregnancy, particularly in the 3rd trimester. (Carpenter MW, Coasting DR, 1982)

Sign and symptoms of diabetics

Following sign and symptoms can occur in diabetics:

For type-1 diabetics:

- extreme thirst
- frequent urination
- sudden unexplained weight loss
- extreme fatigue
- blurred vision
- muscle cramps
- nausea
- vomiting
- constant hunger

For type-2 diabetics:

- increased thirst
- frequent urination
- feeling tired and lethargic
- always feeling hungry
- having cuts that heal slowly
- itching
- skin infections
- blurred vision
- gradually putting on weight
- mood swings
- headaches
- feeling dizzy

> leg cramps

Pancreas – insulin and glucagon secreting organ

The pancreas is a glandular organ that secretes digestive enzymes (internal secretions) and hormones (external secretions). In humans, the pancreas is a yellowish organ about 7 inches (17.8 cm) long and 1.5 inches. (3.8 cm) wide. The pancreas lies beneath the stomach and is connected to the small intestine at the duodenum. The pancreas contains enzyme-producing cells that secrete mainly two hormones. These two hormones are insulin secreted by β-cell and glucagon secreted by alpha-cell. Insulin and glucagon are secreted directly into the bloodstream, and together, they regulate the level of glucose in the blood. Insulin lowers the blood sugar level and increases the amount of glucagon (stored carbohydrate) in the liver. Glucagon slowly increases the blood sugar level if it falls too low. If the insulin secreting cells do not work properly, diabetes occurs. In addition, at least one other type of cell, the pp cells, is present in small numbers in the islets and secrets a hormone of uncertain function called pancreatic polypeptide. (Source: wikipedia the free encyclopedia, April 2008)

The pancreas produces the body's most important enzymes. The enzymes are designed to digest foods and break down starches. The pancreas also helps neutralize chyme and helps break down proteins, fats and starch. Chyme is a thick semi fluid mass of partly digested food that is passed from the stomach to the duodenum. If the pancreas is not working properly to neutralize chyme and break down proteins, fats and starch, starvation may occur.

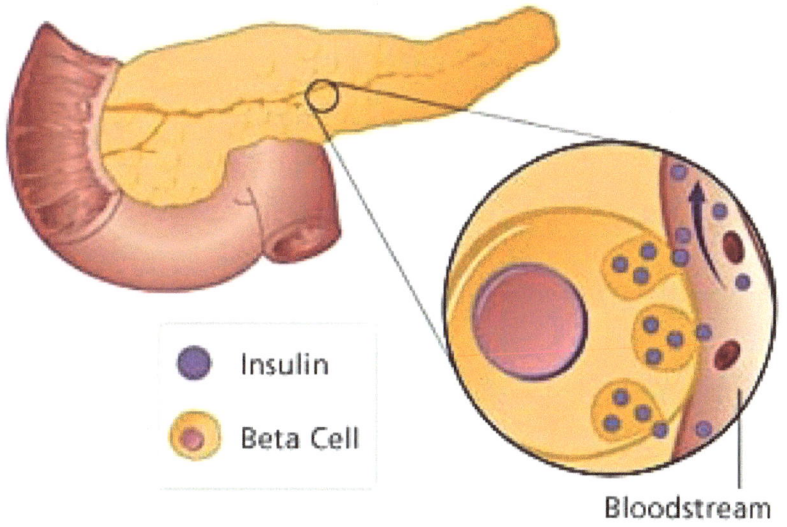

● Insulin

◉ Beta Cell

Bloodstream

Fig: Human Pancreas and its insulin secreting beta cell

The pancreas is composed of two major types of tissues– a) the acini, which secret digestive juices into the duodenum and b) the islets of Langerhans, which do not have any means for emptying their secretions externally but instead, secrete insulin and glucagon directly into the blood.

The pancreas of the human being has 1 to 2 million islets of Langerhans, each only about 0.3 millimeter in diameter and organized around small capillaries into which it's cells secret their hormones. The islets contain three major types of cells,α β and δ cells, which are distinguished from one another by their morphologic and staining characteristics. The β-cells constituting about 60% of all the cells, lie mainly in the middle of each islet and secrete insulin. The α-cells, about 25% of the total, secrete glucagons. And δ-cells, about 10% of the total, secrete somatostatin. The dose interrelations among these cell types in the islets of Langherhans allow direct control of secretion of some of the hormones by the other hormones. For instance, insulin inhibits glucagon secretion and somatostatin inhibits the secretion of both insulin and glucagon. (Guyton, 2000)

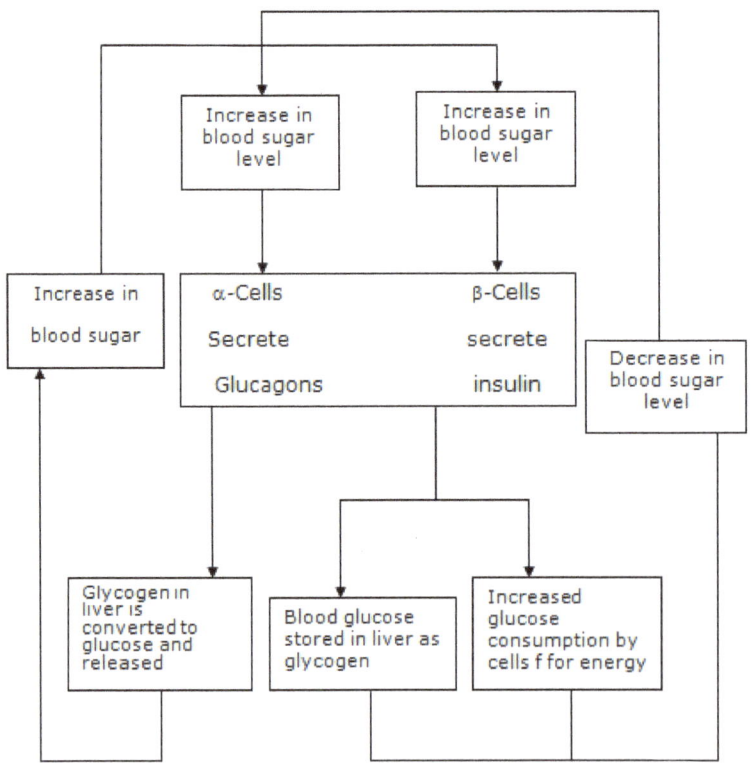

Figure: Regulation of the secretion of insulin and glucagons (Tortora, 1981)

Insulin and diabetes mellitus

Virtually all forms of diabetes mellitus are due to either a decrease in the circulating concentration of insulin (insulin deficiency) or a decrease in the response of peripheral tissues to insulin (insulin resistance) in association with an excess of hormones with actions opposite to those of insulin (glucagons, growth hormone, cortisol and catecholamine). Insulin was first isolated form the pancreas in 1922 by Banting and Best. Historically, insulin has been associated with "blood sugar", and true enough insulin has profound effects on carbohydrate metabolism. Yet its abnormalities of fat metabolism, causing such conditions as acidosis and arteriosclerosis, which are the usual causes of death of a diabetic patient.

Also, in patients with prolonged diabetes, diminished ability to synthesize proteins leads to wasting of the tissues as well as many cellular function disorders. Therefore, it is clear that insulin affects fat and protein metabolism almost as much as it does to the carbohydrate metabolism.

Insulin is a small protein; human insulin has a molecular weight of 5808. It is composed of two amino acid chains, connected to each other by disulfide linkages. When the two amino acid chains are split apart, the functional activity of the insulin molecule is lost. (Guyton, 2000)

Insulin lowers blood-glucose level through the following way; (Khan, 1994)

Insulin causes-   In the liver

1. Increase glycogenesis (Glucose to glycogen)

2. Decrease glycogenolysis (Glycogen to glucose)

3. Decrease neoglucogenesis (glucose from non –

   Carbohydrate sources)

4. Increase uptake of glucose from blood

5. Increase conversion of glucose into fatty acid

In the peripheral tissue (e.g., muscles)

1. Increase glucose transport

2. Increase utilization of glucose (glycolysis)

3. Increase glycogenesis

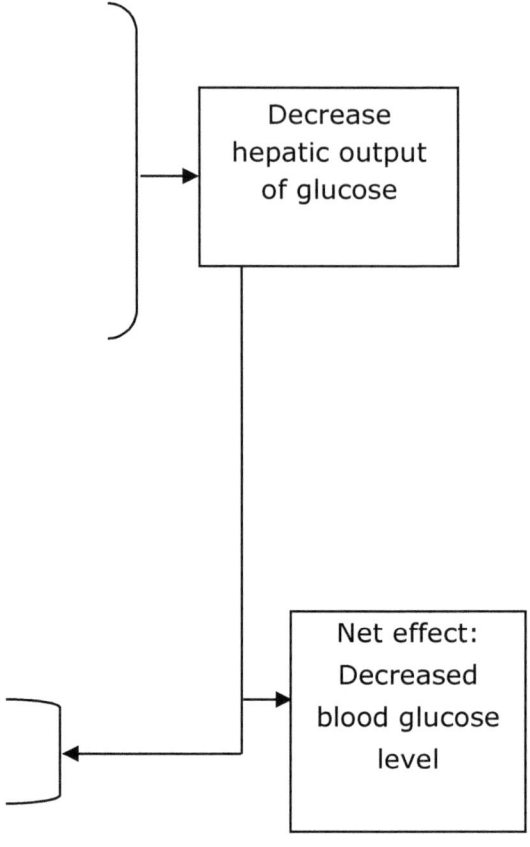

Stimulators	Inhibitors

Glucose Mannose Aminoacids (leucine,arginine and others) Intestinal hormones (GIP, gastrin, secretin, CCK and others) β-ketoacids Acetylcholine Glucagon Cyclic AMP and various cyclic AMP generating substances β-adrenergic stimulating agents Theophylline Sulphonylurease	Somatostatin 2- Deoxy glucose Mannoheptulose α-adrenergic stimulating agents (epinephrine, norepinephrine) β -adrenergic blocking agents (propanolol). Diazoxide Thiazide diuretics K+ depletion phenytoin Alloxan Microtuble inhibitors Streptozotocin

Table: Factors affecting insulin secretion

Increase (anabolic effect)	Decrease(anti catabolic effect)
Carbohydrate metabolism: Glucose transport (muscle adipose tissue) Glucose phosphorylation Glycognesis Glycolysis Pyruvate dehydrogenase activity Pentose Phosphate shunt	Gluconeogenesis Glycogenolysis
Lipid metabolism: Trygleceride synthesis Fatty acid synthesis (liver) Lipoprotein lipase activity (adipose tissue)	Lipolysis Lipoprotein lipase (muscle) Ketogenesis Fattyacid oxidation (liver)
Protein metabolism: Amino acid transport Protein synthesis	Protein degradation

Table: Metabolic actions of Insulin

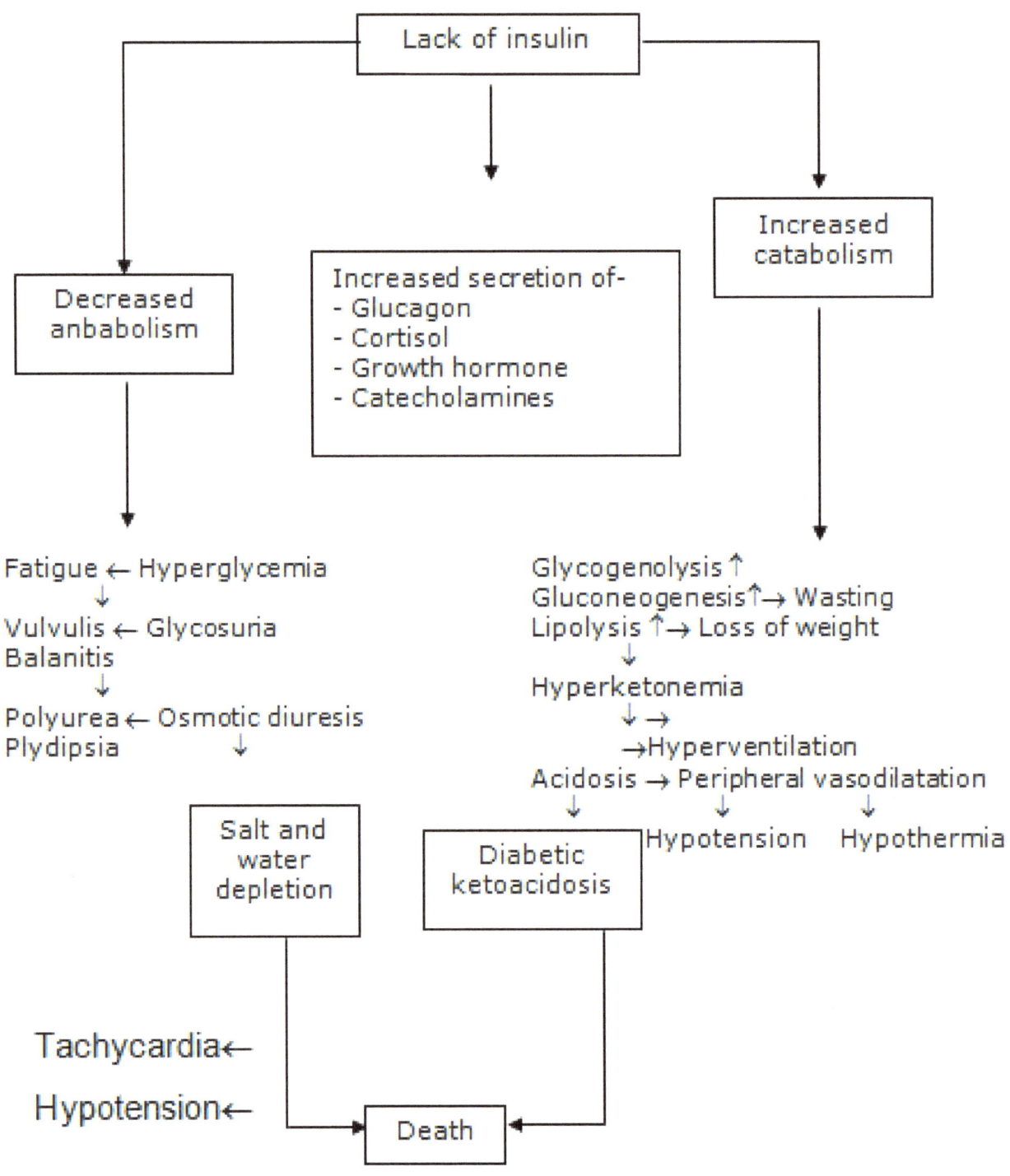

Figure : Pathophysiological basis of symptoms and signs of untreated or uncontrolled diabetes mellitus (Frier and Fisher, 1999)

Drugs used in diabetes and their basic mechanism, how to work the drugs.

With the introduction of insulin, oral anti-diabetic drugs and antibiotics, diabetes is no longer a dreadful disease, and with proper management with diet, drug and exercise a diabetic can enjoy an almost normal life. The etiology of this condition however is still obscure although it definitely has a hereditary tendency. (Satoskar, 2005)

1. Insulin Treatment

Insulin is the mainstay for treatment of diabetes, virtually all type-I and many type-II diabetic patients. Its mode of action can be described as follows-

- ➢ Insulin decreases the intracellular concentration of cAMP by inhibiting enzyme adenylyl cyclase and stimulating phosphodiesterase. So protein kinase is not activated due to absence of cAMP and consequently break down of glycogen is inhibited.
- ➢ Insulin also reduces the sensitivity of protein kinase to cAMP and glycogen synthesis is enhanced.
- ➢ Insulin enhances facilitated diffusion of glucose and activates transport of amino acids to cells.
- ➢ Insulin promotes K^+ and Mg^{++} uptake into cells which may act as "second messenger" to mediate the actions of insulin (Ronald and Shechter, 1991)
- ➢ Insulin can be extracted from porcine and bovine pancreases. Increasingly, 'human' insulin (Humulin) is used, usually made by recombinant DNA technology. It is destroyed in the gastrointestinal tract, and must be given parenterally, usually subscutaneously, but intravenously or occasionally, intramuscularly in emergencies (Rang, 2005)

Different formulations of insulin differ in their duration of action. (Rang, 2005)

- ➢ Fast and short acting soluble insulin: Peak action: 2-4 hours after subcutaneous dose: Duration: 6-8 hours. It can be given intravenously.

- ➢ Intermediate acting: e.g., isophane insulin. It can be mixed with soluble insulin.

- ➢ Long acting: e.g., insulin zinc suspension.

Intranasal and inhalation routes of administration are being investigated. Once in the blood, insulin has a $t_{1/2}$ of about 10 minutes. It is inactivated enzymetically in the liver and kidney, and 10% excreted in the urine. Renal impairment reduces insulin requirement.

The main undesirable effect of insulin is hypoglycemia. This is common and causes brain damage. Allergy to insulin is unusual but may take the form of local or systemic reactions. Severe insulin resistances as a consequence of antibody formation are rare.

2. Oral hypoglycemic agents (Satoskar, 2005) Oral hypoglycemic drugs can often lower blood sugar levels adequately in patient with type 2 diabetes. However, they are not effective in type 1 diabetes. There are several types of oral hypoglycemic agents. The currently available oral anti-diabetic agents are classified according to their predominant mechanism of action:

Stimulators of β-cells, e.g., sulfonylureas.

I.   Inhibitors of gluconeogenesis, e.g., biguanides.

II.   Inhibitors of intestinal α-glucosidases, e.g., acarbose, and

III.   Drugs, which reduces insulin resistance, e.g., glitazones.

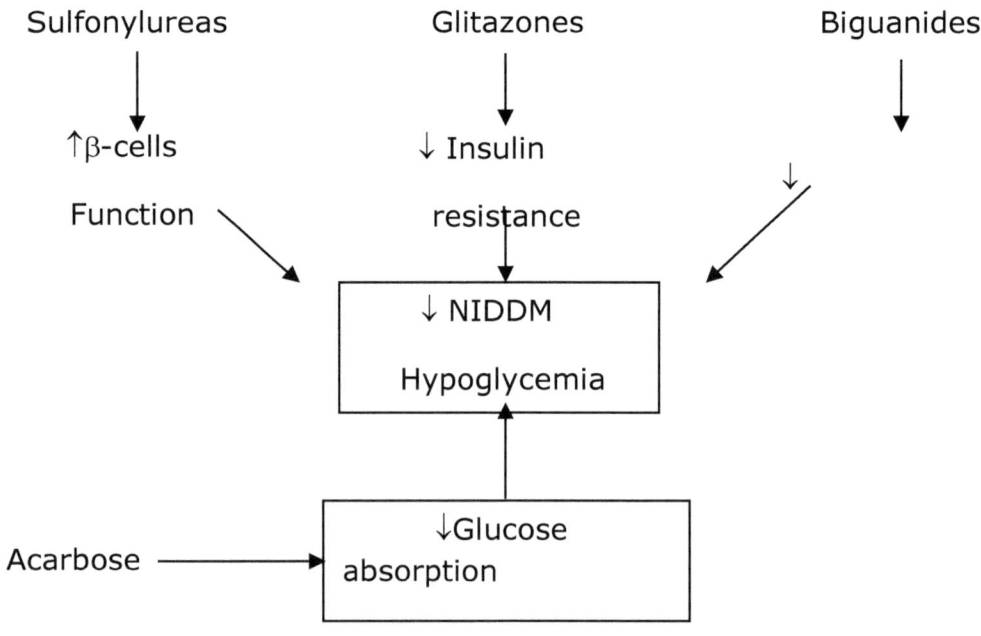

Figure 1.4: Mechanism of action of oral antidiabetic drugs (Satoskar, 1999).

Sulfonylureas

These compounds are chemically related to sulfonamides and have a basic structure as follows: (Satoskar, 1999)

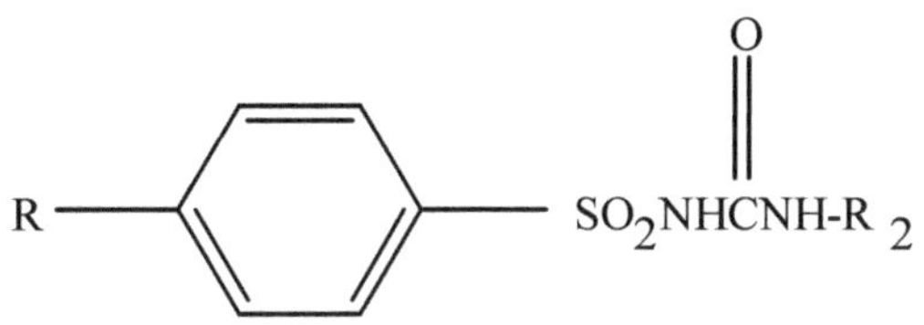

Figure 1.5: General structure of sulfonylureas

The principal effect of suylfonylureas is mediated through stimulation of the release of insulin from the pancreatic β-Cell, but also exert extra pancreatic effects, particularly in hepatic release of glucose (Frier and Fisher, 1999).

Tolbutamide, Chlorpropamide, tolazamide, acetohexamide are belongs to this class. Other three potent sulfonylureas compounds; glyburide (glibenclamide), glipizide and glimepride are considered "Second-generation" hypoglycemic agents.

Sulfonylureas are well absorbed after oral administration and most reach peak plasma concentrations within 2-4 hours.

The sulfonylureas are well tolerated. The important toxic effects are hypoglycemia, allergic skin rash and bone marrow depression (Rang, 1999).

Biguanides

A free guanidine radical is though to be essential for the hypoglycemic effect of biguandies (Satoskar, 1999).

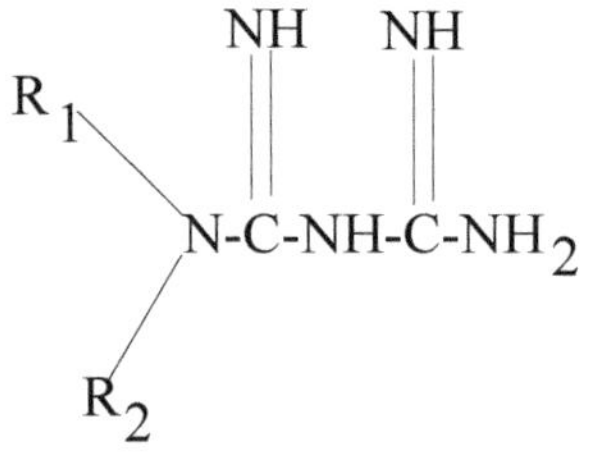

$$
\begin{array}{c}
\quad\quad\quad NH \quad\quad NH \\
R_1 \quad\quad \| \quad\quad \| \\
\quad\quad N\text{-}C\text{-}NH\text{-}C\text{-}NH_2 \\
R_2
\end{array}
$$

Figure 1.6: General structure of biguandies

These are orally active hypoglycemic agents that do not require functioning β-cells. Their action is complex and incompletely understood. They increase glucose uptake in skeletal muscle and have effects on glucose abosrption and hepatic glucose production. Biguandies commonly produce and unpleasant, better or metallic taste, anorexia, muscular weakness and as excessive weight loss on some patients. Rarely, anaphylactic shock or generalized urticaria can occur (Rang, 1999).

α-glucosidase inhibitors

Acarbose, an inhibitor of intestinal α-glucosidase is used in type-2 patients inadequately controlled by diet with or without other agents. It delays carbohydrate absorption reducing the postprandial increase in blood glucose. The commonest adverse effects are its main action and consist of flatulence, loose stools or diarrhea and abdominal pain and bloating (Rang, 1999).

Potential new anti-diabetic drugs or glitazones

Several agents are currently being studied including $α_2$-antagonists, inhibitors of fatty acid oxidation and agents that enhance the response of tissue to insulin notably the thiazolidinediones e.g., troglitazone (Rang, 1999).

In vitro diabetic model for testing antidiabetic effects of plants (Soumpanath A. 2005)

Anti-diabetic effects of plants can be assessed clinically in humans, in vivo using animal models or in vitro using a variety of test systems. Each level of testing has its advantages and limitations. Human studies are ultimately necessary because the product is tested by intended route in the eventually beneficiary of an effective treatment. However, in many cases it is neither feasible nor ethical to conduct initial trials in human because little is known about the safety or efficacy of the verb or even of a suitable does or method of preparation. It is therefore appropriate to conduct studies in animals prior to administering the herb to humans.

Preliminary testing of herb in an animal model can give valuable information on the type of extract to be made, a suitable does, likely toxic effects, and of course efficacy of a herb or its components, when used clinically.

In vitro tests can play an important role in the evaluation of anti-diabetic or other medicinal plants, as initial screening tools or as follow-up to human to human or animal studies. Biological materials used in theses includes, in increasing order of simplicity perused whole organs, isolated tissues, cells in primary or immortal culture, sub cellular membranes or purified receptors, and enzymes.

Rationale behind the in vitro models used in diabetic research

A rang of in vitro models are available to study potential antidiabetic activity in plant extracts. They are based on the primary need to control hyperglycemia in diabetes and the various means of achieving goal. In vitro models may be used to screen randomly or ethnobotanically selected materials for a specific activity that would result in the lowering of blood glucose levels.

It is relevant in the context of in vitro testes for antidiabetic activity to examine the source and fate of glucose in the body in the normal and diabetic states. Glucose is derived primarily from the digestion of dietary carbohydrates in the gastrointestinal tract, from which it is absorbed into the blood by passive and active mechanisms. In the fed state, a rise in blood glucose normally stimulates insulin secretion from the pancreas. This hormone initiates glucose uptake into specific target tissues, primarily in liver, muscle, and fat cells (adipocytes). It promotes glucose oxidation and glycogen deposition in liver and muscle and the incorporation of glucose (as glycerol) into triglycerides in adipocytes. These combined activities have the effect of lowering elevated plasma glucose resulting from the intake of a meal. In the fasted state, glucose and insulin levels decrease. Glucose is then mobilized from glycogen stores in the liver (glycogenolysis).

Another important source of glucose in the fasted state is gluconegenesis the de novo formation of glucose from smaller non sugar, precursor molecules. This occurs in the liver and to a lesser extent kidneys and is under the control of glucagons, a counter-hormone whose levels rise as those of insulin fall and vice versa. When glucagons levels are high and those of insulin are low, gluconeogenesis and glycogenolysis are stimulated and glucose enters the bloodstream.

In diabetes, insulin is absent (type-1) or insufficient (Type-2). In type-2 diabetes, insulin target tissues re generally less responsive to insulin (insulin resistant) than normal. The fine balance between glucose uptake into garget organs and release of hepatic glucose is impaired, resulting in abnormally high fasting glucose levels as well as poor glucose tolerance following meal.

From the foregoing, the following mechanisms have been proposed for an agent that would lower or control plasma glucose levels;

Inhibition of carbohydrate-digesting enzymes, reducing amount of route of glucose release from diet.

Impairment of glucose uptake from the small intestine.

Stimulation of insulin secretion from the small intestine.

Insulinomimetic or insulin-sensitizing activity at insulin target tissues i.e., liver, skeletal muscle or adipocytes.

Antagonism of glucagons activity.

For cure the diabetic you can use that medicine. That are FDA approved very good working drugs. Doctors are recommends that medicine form very early of modern treatment.

Impact of vitamins in diabetics

Generally there is no impact of vitamin in diabetics. Diabetic is a metabolic disorder. There is no relation with vitamin. But recently a research show that deficiency of vitamin D will increase of type -1 and type -2 diabetics. Deficiency of vitamin D can increase cardio vascular diseases also.

Yoga and Diabetics

Yoga is most popular for prevention of many desies. Yoga have some positive effect on diabetics. Yoga have effect on both type of diabetic type1 and type 2 diabetics. Main mechanism of action of yoga on diabetics is increase the glucose uptake and use of glucose. In one reasurce says excessive physical exercise can cause hypoglycemia and cause to death. So we have to concern about that.

Some weight loss programmes help in reducing diabates such as this listed below :

Weight Watchers Products

Weight Watchers produces many of its own products to help you with your weight loss goals. They offer many recipes online along with many simple articles and publications to teach you how to be healthy and eat healthy as well as fitness tips.

Weight Watchers creates many of its own meals. It has many full meals as well as deserts. You can buy anything from yogurt to cheese, to bread in its store. They also sell books and magazines that will give you more recipes and show you how to get started with the program.

On top of the many products you can buy from Weight Watchers themselves there are also many products, which they have endorsed. These include certain brands, which produce everything from popcorn, soup, vegetables and Jell-o to vegetarian meals.

Reviews

Many of the users of this program say that it works very well. You just have to make sure you do the work. That means that when do your best to stick to the program it will work for you and you will lose weight. A lot of people think this is one of the best weight loss plans they know of or have tried.

The negatives that many people report tend to be about the online version of Weight Watchers. You have the choice of joining the regular program that asks you to join a group and attend meetings. If you join the online website, you do not have to attend meetings however there are many drawbacks. When you go online, you are not getting very much for your money. You also will need to sign into the website every day to keep track of what you're eating and how you're doing on the plan. For many people this is difficult.

Benefits

There are many benefits to the Weight Watchers program. This program gives you a lot of support because you are encouraged to attend weekly meetings with others who are working on the same thing you are as well as being able to talk with professionals and those who have completed the program successfully. This way you are able to motivate each other and get through the process. You are also given many tools, which include cookbooks, meal plans, work out plans, and many other tools, which you can use right from your mobile phone.

Weight Watchers also uses weigh ins so that you can see how you are doing compared to your goal. These weigh ins are confidential so that you don't have to worry about anyone else knowing your weight. Finally, Weight Watchers counts the calories for you so that you don't have to worry about it and can simply eat your meals based on the point values.

Risks

There are numerous problems that can arise as a result of Weight Watchers. One of these is vitamin deficiency. Users of this plan have to follow a point system which does not take into consideration any vitamins or minerals. This means that most people may not eat the proper amount of vitamins that they need in a day because they are only eating based on fat, protein, carbs and fiber.

Another problem with Weight Watchers is that you don't count the calories you consume. The program allows you to eat anything you want so long as you stay within your target points for the day. That means you could end up eating very few calories. Everyone needs a certain number of calories to survive and with this program a lot of people don't meet that number therefore undernourishment is a very real possibility.

The third and final problem with this plan is sodium. The average person is supposed to consume only 2300 mg of sodium per day. Any more than this can cause many problems. If you are eating Weight Watchers meals for every meal of the day then you will be consuming far more sodium than recommended.

There are a few different risks that could happen if you choose to follow this diet. However, it is also a beneficial plan. So look at the risks and benefits and decide what's best for you.

Conclusion

A diabetic is a metabolic disorder. It can cause by genetically, auto immune disorder, side effect of some drug and by food habit. Hyperglycemia and Hypoglycemia both are very bad for health. So everyone should take steps when they will affected on diabetics. All of us have to know the sign and symptoms of diabetics. We have to know also what we have to know after effected on diabetics.

Author .. T. Harry

Editor… O. Dave